How Austin Got His Muscles

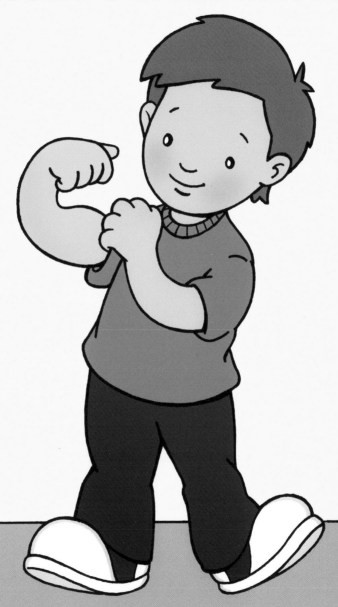

Shari Bilt Boockvar, M.S., R.D.

Illustrated by Kathy Kerber

AuthorHouse™
1663 Liberty Drive
Bloomington, IN 47403
www.authorhouse.com
Phone: 1-800-839-8640

First published by AuthorHouse 8/28/2009

ISBN: 978-1-4389-8054-6 (sc)

Library of Congress Control Number: 2009908543

Printed in the United States of America
Bloomington, Indiana

This book is printed on acid-free paper.

authorHOUSE®

To the two "apples of my eyes,"
my son Austin and husband Peter

This is Austin.
He does the same things that you do.
He goes to school and plays in the playground when the weather is nice.

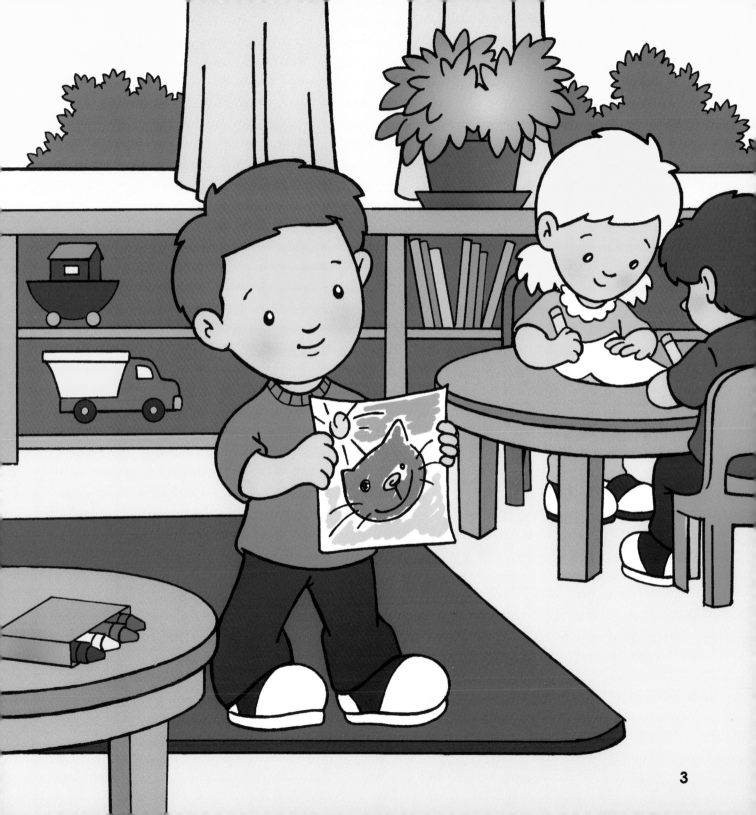

After school,
Austin plays in the snow during the winter and plays all kinds of sports in the spring, summer, and fall. For all these things,
Austin needs his muscles!

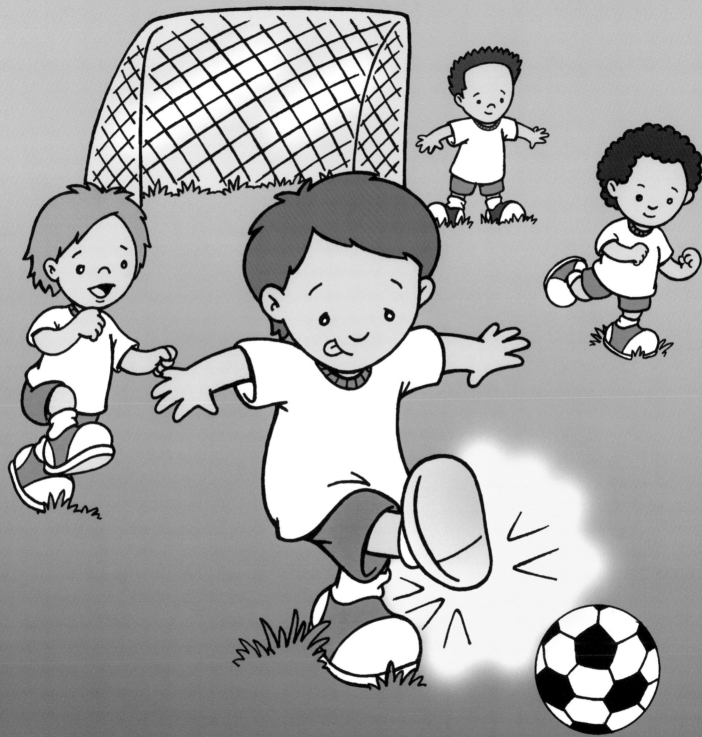

Every day, Austin likes to help his mommy make his meals.
But there is one problem ...

He always wants to eat his dessert *first!*
At every meal, Austin asks for his dessert right away.

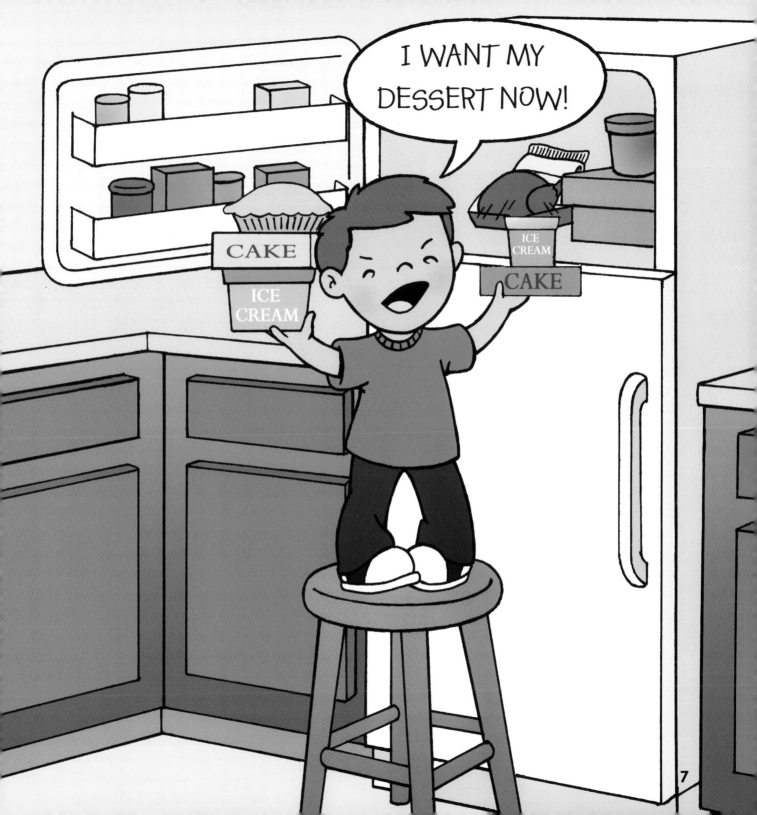

At breakfast,
Austin asks for dessert first.

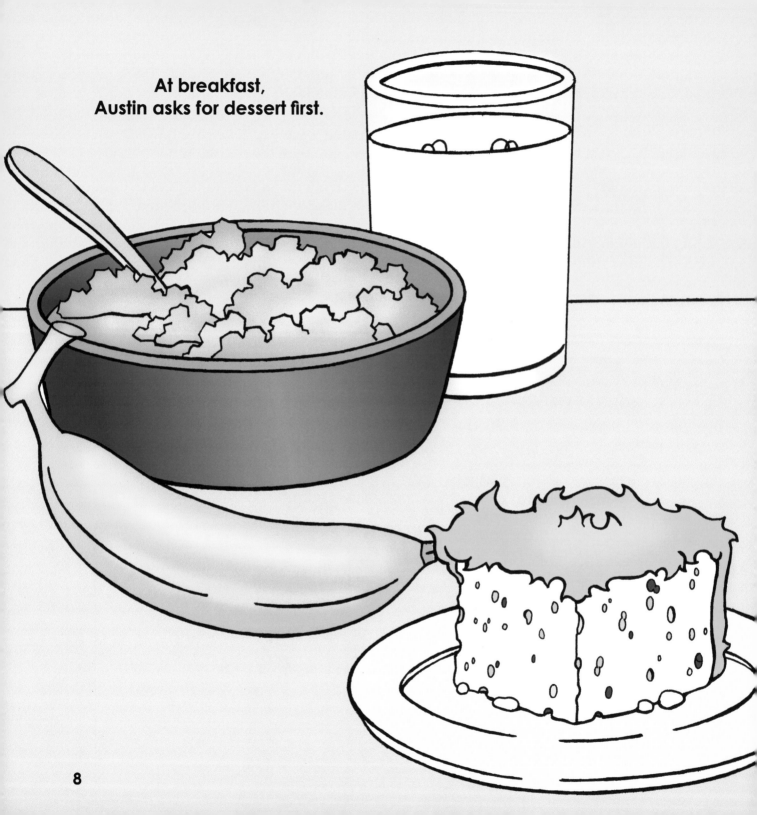

At lunch,
Austin craves dessert first.

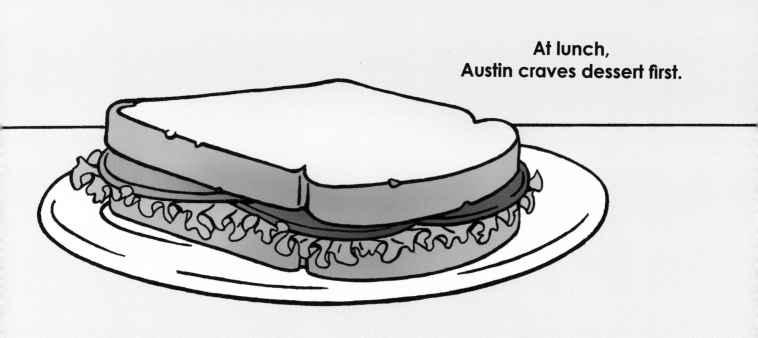

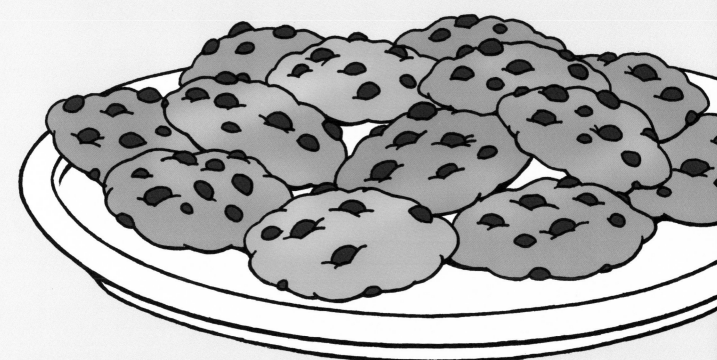

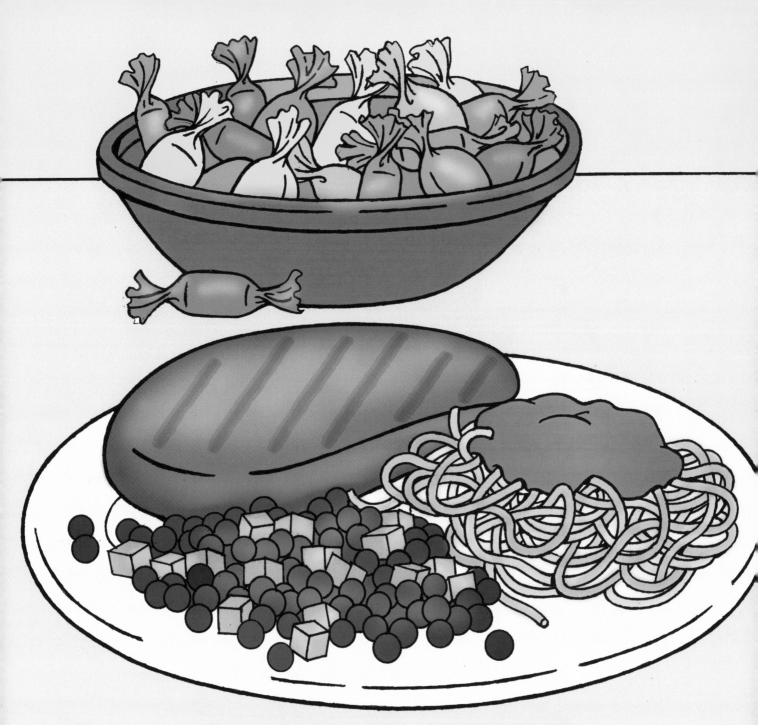

He even hopes to eat his dessert for dinner!

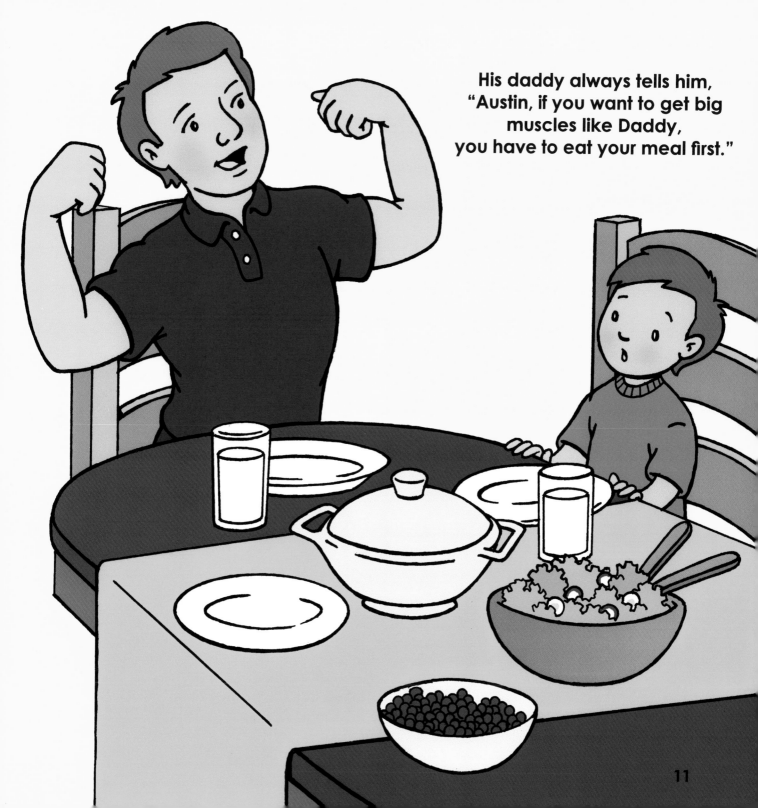

His daddy always tells him,
"Austin, if you want to get big
muscles like Daddy,
you have to eat your meal first."

11

His mommy always says to him,
"Austin, eating dessert first is not going to make you big and strong."
So Austin, Mommy, and Daddy make a deal.

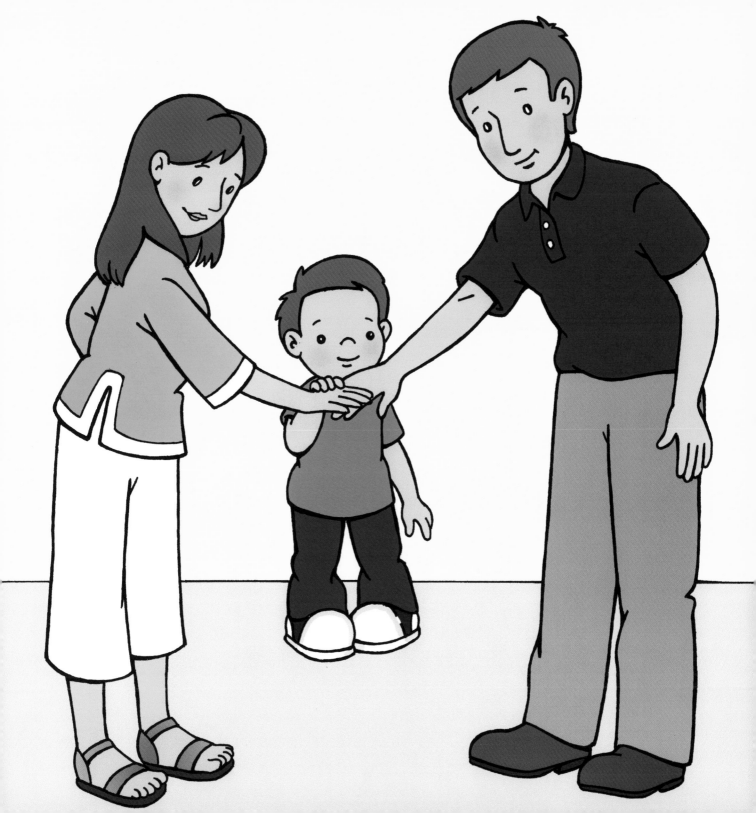

If Austin can finish his breakfast, lunch, and dinner,
he can have a special treat every night! But there is one catch ...

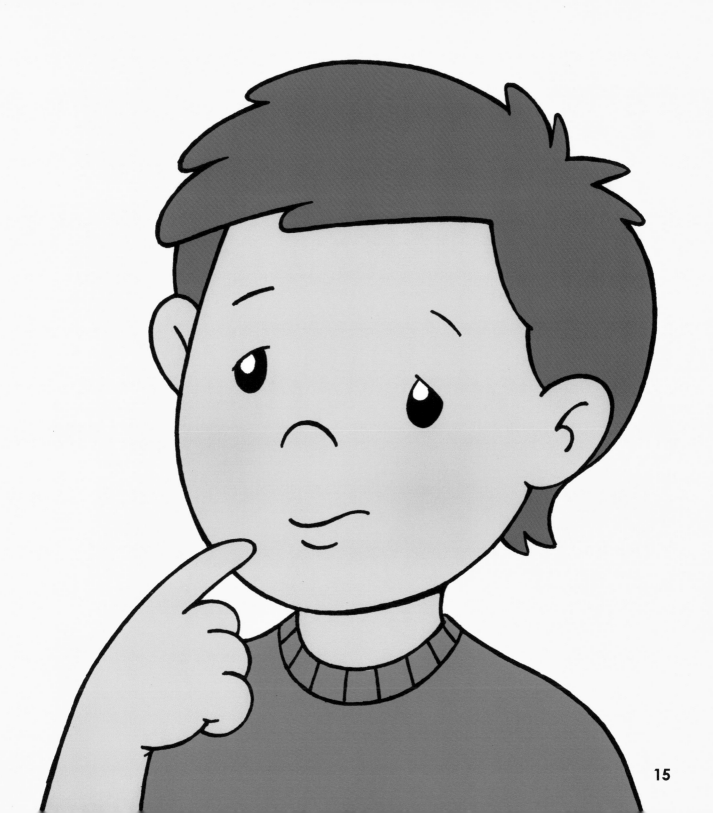

He has to pick a fruit or vegetable
that is one of the colors of the rainbow to eat with each meal.
Mommy tells him eating lots of different colored foods will help give him
lots of energy and big muscles to better play all his sports and games.

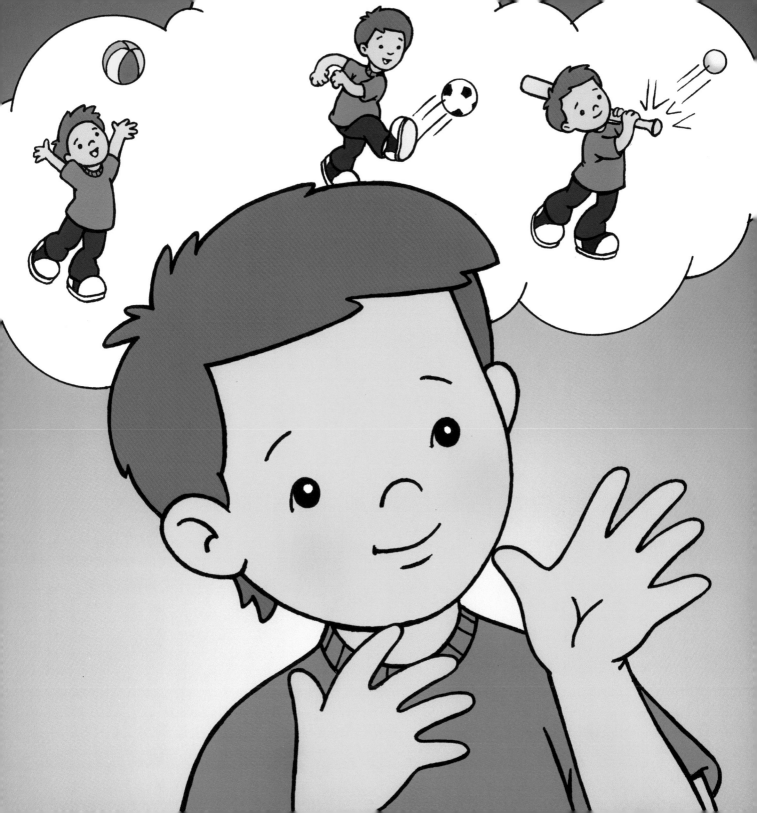

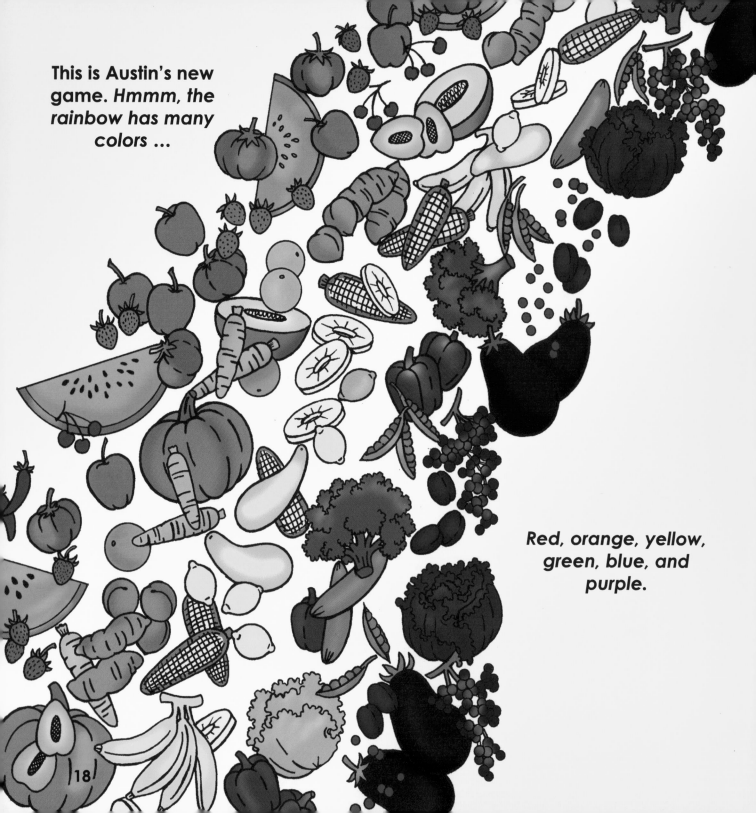

This is Austin's new game. *Hmmm, the rainbow has many colors ...*

Red, orange, yellow, green, blue, and purple.

18

At breakfast, he chooses different colored foods for his meals:

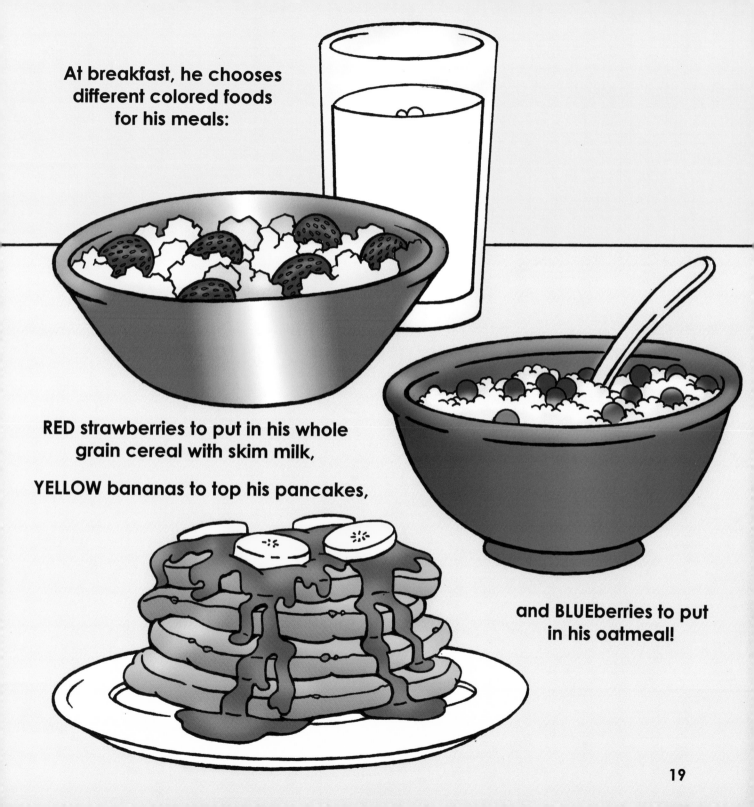

RED strawberries to put in his whole grain cereal with skim milk,

YELLOW bananas to top his pancakes,

and BLUEberries to put in his oatmeal!

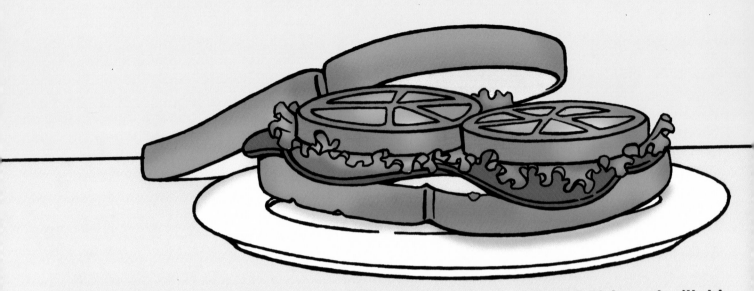

At lunch, he chooses RED tomatoes for his sandwich, ORANGES to eat with his chicken fingers, and sometimes GREEN beans and YELLOW zucchini with dip!

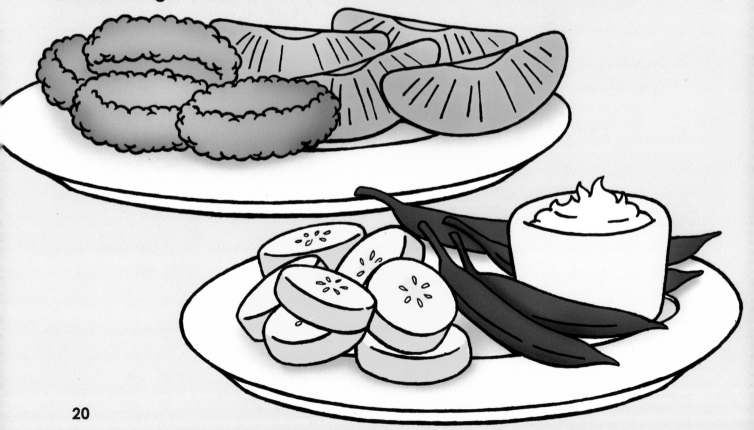

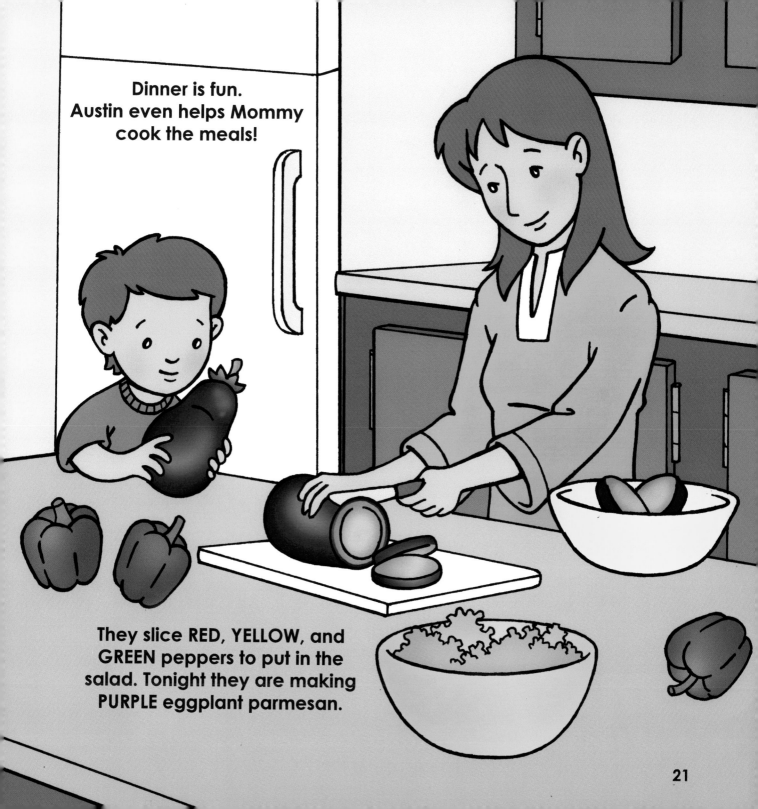

Dinner is fun.
Austin even helps Mommy
cook the meals!

They slice RED, YELLOW, and
GREEN peppers to put in the
salad. Tonight they are making
PURPLE eggplant parmesan.

21

Austin does such a good job of eating his rainbow meals that he always gets to choose his *favorite* dessert ...

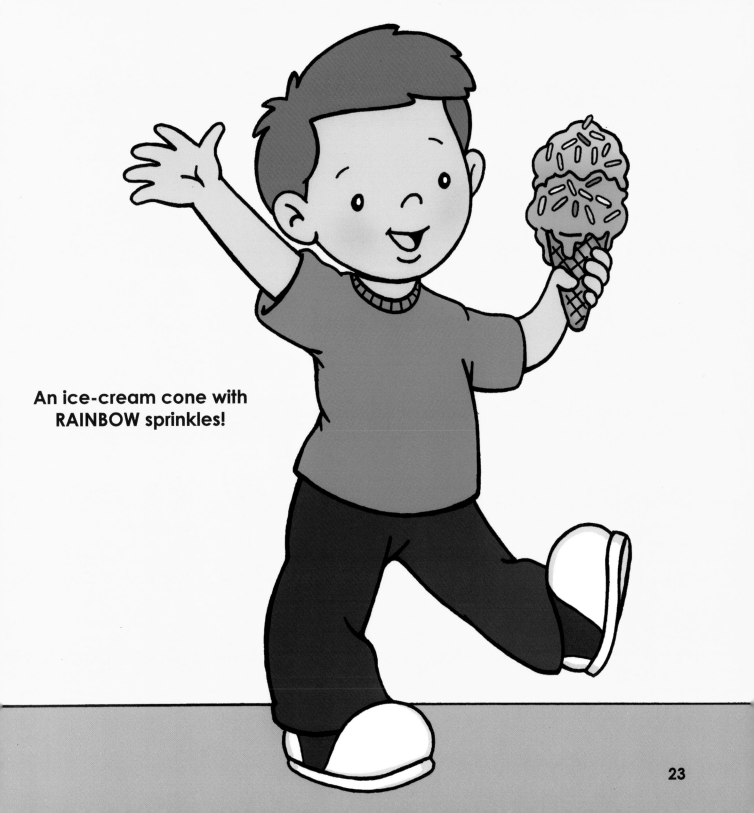

An ice-cream cone with
RAINBOW sprinkles!

23

And guess what Austin has now ...

Lots of energy to play and *big muscles!*

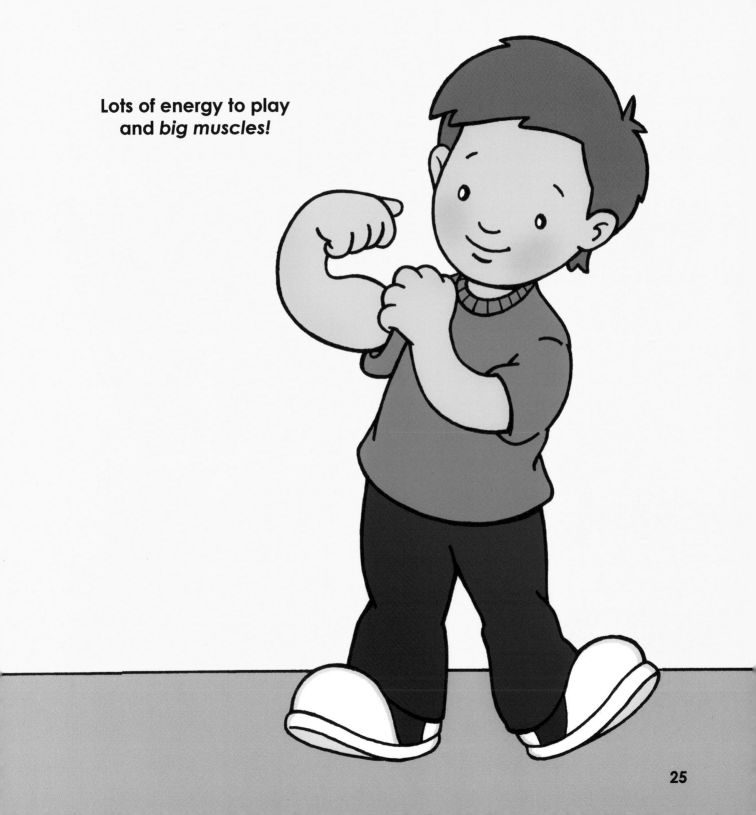

FOODS IN THE COLORS OF THE RAINBOW

Red (good for your heart and memory): Strawberries, Apples, Cherries, Tomatoes, Raspberries, Beets, Red Peppers, Watermelon

Orange (good for your eyes, bones, and skin): Carrots, Oranges, Cantaloupe, Sweet Potatoes, Apricots, Pumpkin, Peaches, Papaya

Yellow (good for your teeth, gums, and can heal cuts): Bananas, Squash, Corn, Lemons, Mangoes, Pineapple

Green (good for your bones, eyes, and teeth): Broccoli, Green Beans, Green Peppers, Spinach, Dark-Green Lettuces, Brussels Sprouts, Asparagus, Artichokes, Avocado, Kiwi, Peas, Cucumber, Celery

Blue/Purple (good for your heart and brain): Blueberries, Eggplant, Grapes, Blackberries, Figs, Purple Cabbage, Plums

OTHER IDEAS YOU CAN TRY

1. Try one new colorful fruit or vegetable this week that you have never tasted before.

2. Cook a new recipe that has at least two colorful fruits or vegetables.

3. Plant a mini fruit or vegetable garden.

4. Purchase **BROWN** whole-grain foods (look for those with 3–5 grams of fiber per serving).

5. Eat or drink **WHITE** low-fat dairy foods such as 1 percent or skim milk, cheese, yogurt, and cottage cheese (look for those with no more than 3 grams of fat per serving).